THE DAY WITH YOGA

Inspirational Words to Guide Daily Life

Compiled and edited by
Elisabeth Haich

Translated by
D.Q. Stephenson

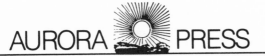

AURORA PRESS

P.O. Box 573   Santa Fe, N.M. 87504

First published in 1983 by:
Aurora Press Inc.
PO Box 573
Santa Fe, N.M. 87504

Email: Aurorep@aol.com

Printed in the U.S.A.
Originally published in German as
Der Tag mit Yoga

Library of Congress Cataloging in Publication Data

The Day with Yoga
   Translation of Der Tag mit Yoga.
   1. Yoga—Quotations, maxims, etc. I. Haich, Elizabeth
B132. Y6T2813   1976   181'.45   76-42208
ISBN 0-943358-12-4

Contents

Elisabeth Haich: The Day with Yoga

Yoga is not a religion; it is crystallized truth.

E. Haich

He is not a man that cannot call one hour of each day his own.

Mosche I öb von Sasow

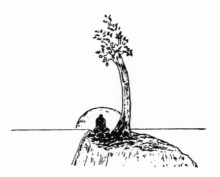

INTRODUCTION

Just as sunlight consists of seven colors and breaks up into these seven colors, so the elemental divine creative power comprises seven creative principles which, working together or apart, constitute constructive—and also destructive—forces in the Universe. Everything in existence was and is created by these forces: heavenly bodies like the sun and the planets, or plants, animals and human beings. It was these forces that also created the planets, that work in them and out of them, and so men called these forces after the planets, bestowing upon each the name of the planet in and out of which it operates most potently and to which it imparts its characteristics. Even today, for instance, we call the power operating most strongly in the sun and characterizing its vibrations solar power, and the emanations from the moon lunar power, and so forth. Each takes its name from the heavenly body whose emanations it characterizes.

These seven creative principles operate not only together but also separately, not only in space but also in time. From time immemorial men have noticed that the vibrations in the earth's atmosphere are not immutable. They discovered that these operative energies alternate at certain times in a particular rhythm. These alternations were so noticeable and striking that men divided and named time according to these alternating and rhythmically recurrent periods. And since men called the creative principles after the planets, they called the seven consecutive days after the planets too. Thus the day when the vibrations of the sun are strongest has become Sunday. The day of the moon became Monday and the names of the days of the week are all similarly named after the various planets. Thus the week came into being.

In English the days were named not after the gods of Roman mythology which symbolize the seven elemental forces but after the gods of Teutonic mythology. However, the names are the same as far as their meaning is concerned. Sunday was named after the sun, Monday after the moon, Tuesday after the god Tiw, who is identical with Mars the Roman god of war, Wednesday after the god Woden, the counterpart of the Roman Mercury, Thursday after the god Thor, who is identical with the Roman Jupiter, Friday after the goddess Freia, who is identical with the Roman goddess Venus, and Saturday after the Roman Saturn.

In Indian philosophy these natural forces operating secretly in the earth's atmosphere are called Tatvas. Indians adapt their whole life to these forces—the Tatvas. They try to bring all the important events of their lives into harmony with the Tatvas. Knowing what different Tatvas are operative in turn in the various parts of the day—morning, midday, evening and night—they even go so far as to divide up their day accordingly. Of course, these Tatvas are considerably less potent than the main Tatvas which are at work throughout the day.

If the Tatvas operating on a particular day were unfavorable, an Indian would never think of embarking on anything important, whether it was contracting a marriage, starting a business, going on a journey or anything else. He knows that such an undertaking would be doomed to failure. One often hears of Western businessmen in India who cannot understand why Indians sometimes postpone pressing business discussions, the signing of important and often very urgent contracts, supplies of goods and the like. The Indians know why! They have found out which Tatvas are active on these days, and if the prevailing Tatvas are not in harmony with these affairs, they postpone the completion of the business to a time when the right Tatvas, that is, those suited to the matter, are active.

A different creative energy is at work on each day of the week. Nature and all living creatures, be it plants, animals or human beings, are influenced by these vibrations, and bathe and float in the power operating in Nature on that day.

Plants and animals obey these vibrations automatically. To some extent the same might be said of human beings. But through the operation of their intelligence they have drawn very far away from Nature and its rhythm. For instance, they no longer go to bed when the sun sets as animals do, they no longer comply with their instincts; instead they have brought their whole life and its rhythm into conformity with what their intelligence reveals to them. Thus man gradually became more and more divorced from Nature and hence from natural forces. It very often happens that these work against man. No wonder, then, that men are no longer familiar with the forces of Nature, no longer master and possess them, and must consequently suffer from physical and spiritual disease.

All the great teachers of mankind have shown that man has the power to bend these forces to his will and to direct them. But man has forgotten that he possesses this ability. And so he must learn through suffering to re-establish contact with these forces in order to be able to master and direct them. One important step in this direction is to recognize the vibrations of the forces operative on the various days of the week and deliberately to attune oneself to them. In doing this we are greatly assisted by the names of the various days, for they tell us on which day we can get to know the particular energy operating then.

But how can we attune ourselves to the various creative vibrations? How can we appropriate them to ourselves and control them? That great temptress, the snake, the understanding, has lured us out of the primal paradisiacal state, and it must therefore help us to tread the weary and narrow path that leads us back into Paradise. We fell out of this heavenly primal state *unconsciously*, and we must return *in full consciousness* of what we are doing in order to recover the primal state and never to lose it again.

This path from the unconscious into the divine self-consciousness is called Yoga.

A very useful Yoga exercise by which to attain this end is to attune ourselves to the vibrations of the day by concentrating on certain thoughts. These thoughts must be selected in such a way that they arouse in us the energy corresponding to the day.

In this little book we have carefully chosen and collected quotations which show us how we can attune ourselves to the vibrations of the day with the help of a thought.

Let us open its pages, say, at Sunday where we shall find the thoughts appropriate to that day, and select a sentence as an aid to concentration. Let us think this thought through and through and attempt to understand it completely. Let us ponder its meaning ever more deeply in order to extract its profoundest sense and meditate upon it. Let us through our inmost understanding appropriate the wisdom it contains and identify ourselves with it. We shall find that what we first take the sentence we concentrate upon to mean is quite different from what we subsequently understand by it in *a state of profound concentration*. Slowly we have become identical with it; that is to say, we have awakened in ourselves the spiritual vibrations latent in the sentence and made them part of ourselves. And in this way we have achieved our aim: we have got to know the vibrations of the day and attuned ourselves to them. We perform this mental Yoga exercise every day, using on Monday the quotations given for Monday, on Tuesday those given for Tuesday, and so forth. On each day we concentrate on one of the quotations. They will reveal to us ever new truths and profundities which were always latent in them; it is simply that we did not realize they were there.

By means of this Yoga exercise we shall be able to attune ourselves to the vibrations of the day, and if we practise every day we shall reach the stage where we shall immediately recognize the vibrations hidden in the quotations. Then there will be nothing to prevent us from recognizing the vibrations of creative energy in the atmosphere of the earth even without the help of the quotations and from *consciously* attuning ourselves to them. To this end we need patience and perseverance, but he who does not relinquish the struggle against ignorance will in the end master the primal forces of creation. Man was endowed with the power to do this when he was created!

ELISABETH HAICH

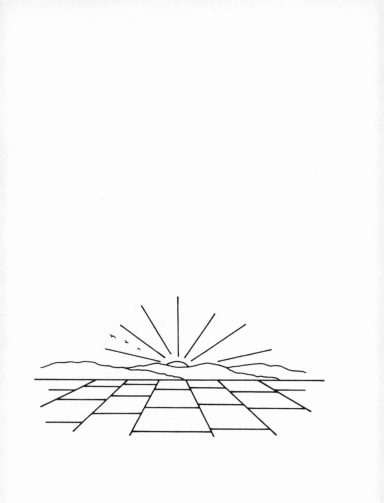

SUNDAY
The Power of the Sun

The power of the sun is the energy of the Divine Self. Just as the sun is the center, ruler and life-giving light of the solar system, radiating its bright effluence in every direction, so, in its manifestation as spiritual light, solar energy brings absolute truth, self-assurance, self-confidence, self-reliance, the power to govern rightly—but also tyranny—love of freedom and radiant health.

The path from unconsciousness to divine self-assurance,
that is Yoga;
The path from slavery to freedom, that is Yoga;
The path from isolation to unity, that is Yoga.

E. Haich

Self-confidence is the cornerstone of life. Remove it and
life will fall apart.

Yesudian

I stand for truth. Truth will never mix with untruth. And
even if the whole world is against me, truth must triumph
in the end.

Vivekananda

Bring light, and evil vanishes in the twinkling of an eye.
Strengthen your character and let your true nature shine
forth, radiant, glorious, ever-pure, and awaken it in
everyone you meet.

Vivekananda

I wish we all entered a state in which we could see the
true self inside even the most wretched of human beings
and, instead of condemning it, say: "Rise, thou radiant
one! Rise, thou eternally pure one! Rise thou who wert
never born and canst never die. Rise, thou almighty one.
Manifest thy true nature!"

Vivekananda

Make all the experiences life can offer part of yourself. Without experiences of your own you will never recognize truth.

Yesudian

Genius is formed in stillness, character in the stream of human life.

Goethe

There are no wicked men, there are only ignorant men! In the presence of a true man the mask of the false man drops.

Ramakrishna

So long as we look at everything from our own point of view, we shall never recognize truth.

Brunton

Say: I am I! And when you say it, feel in your little self the breath of your great self.

Rückert

The more you animate your body, the more conscious you become in your Self.

Yesudian

If we turn the spirit inward, we acquire the power of discernment. Through the power of discernment we find our way to the truth.

Ramakrishna

Only those confined in spirit make the distinction: "This is my friend, and that is my enemy." He who is spiritually free loves them all, just as the sun shines without distinction on noble plants and on weeds.

Lama of Saskya

The light of your true being shines from your center, illuminates your whole body, just as the sun illuminates the whole world from the center of the solar system.

Maharishi

Man does not step from error to truth, but from truth to truth, from a lower to a higher truth.

Vivekananda

The night is far spent, the day is at hand: let us therefore cast off the works of darkness and let us put on the armour of light.

Romans XIII, 12

Everything that weakens you in body, mind, and spirit is a poison. There is no life in it, it cannot be true. The truth strengthens, the truth is purity, the truth is pure knowledge.

Vivekananda

Thou the sun that hidest the truth with thy golden disc, remove the veil that I may see the truth that is in thee; I have recognized the truth that is in thee; I have recognized the true meaning of thy beams and thy glory and have seen what appears in thee. I see the truth in thee, and what is in thee is in me, and I am that I am!

Upanishads

Fortunate art thou! Thou wilt achieve thy goal. Thy race is blessed in thee, for thou strivest to become the eternal by freeing thyself from the bonds of error.

Sankaracharya

You cannot believe in God unless you believe in yourself.

Vivekananda

Never forget that the spirit is king in you! You are spirit, therefore conduct yourself like a king.

Yesudian

The sublime ideal of the Almighty that we have before our eyes shows that we have the same sublimity within us. One day we shall make it reality.

Yesudian

We know what we are but know not what we may be.

Shakespeare

The sun shines not only on the mountain peak but also on the valley. In the same way the spiritual man sheds light in life, his eye sees all, from God down to the creature.

Yesudian

If the truth is on your side, there is no place left for fear.

Yesudian

On earth there is no absolute truth, only partial truths. Only when we have recognized all the partial truths do we find the absolute truth on a spiritual level in ourselves.

E. Haich

Do not cling to old superstitions. Be ever open to new truths.

Vivekananda

Freedom and the highest love must be united; then neither can become a fetter.

Vivekananda

To bear a simple truth often demands a giant's strength, for truth weighs more than anything else in this world.

Yesudian

No word of truth can ever be lost. It may be hidden under weeds for centuries but sooner or later it will come to light. Truth is indestructible. Virtue is indestructible. Purity is indestructible.

Vivekananda

Everything can be sacrificed for truth but truth cannot be sacrificed for anything.

Vivekananda

S
u
n
d
a
y

Truth knows no compromise. Teach truth and never forgive superstition; never pull truth down to the level of the listener.

Vivekananda

To love truth is better than to know it.

Confucius

For with thee is the fountain of life: in thy light shall we see light.

Psalm 36, 9

The true nature of man is perfection. Its conscious expression is perfect health in mind and body. This is happiness.

Yesudian

I must make the highest manifest! I cannot be satisfied with less.

Yesudian

Know ye not that ye are the temple of God, and that the Spirit of God dwelleth in you?

I Corinthians, III, 16

Arise! Awake! What art thou about? If the body is to perish, let it perish in work. To awaken the divine in thyself and in others is the aim.

Vivekananda

If thou believest thou art a body, thou art divided from the universe. If thou believest thou art a spirit, thou art a spark of the eternal fire. If thou believest thou art the divine Self, thou art all things.

Vivekananda

Gold remains gold, whether it tumbles into the ditch or is set on the most holy of altars. Always it remains unchanged. So it is with the man in whom the spirit is awake like the sun at midday. Nothing in this world can defile him, even if he mixes with "publicans and sinners."

Yesudian

Be creative and grow at every step! Death is the creation of a dying mind. Life is the creation of a living mind.

Yesudian

He who has known God sheds all fetters, and along with vanished suffering, he strips off birth and death.

Upanishads

Perfection need not be attained, it is in us already. Immortality and happiness do not have to be acquired for we have them already. They have been ours for all time.

Vivekananda

If you are bound, you will remain bound. If you dare to say that you are free, you are free that very same moment.

Vivekananda

Every spirit is divine according to its nature and ability.

Vivekananda

You offer many means of deliverance! What does that mean? The best deliverance is: presence of the spirit.

Goethe

Once you are in the power of this truthfulness, you will not be able to tell an untruth even in a dream. You will be truthful in thought, word and deed.

Ramakrishna

Unless you are ready to change every minute, you can never recognize the truth. But you must stand firm and persevere in your quest for truth.

Vivekananda

Everything you say will be the truth. You can say to a man: "be blessed!", and he will be blessed. If a man is ill and you say to him: "be well," he will at once be well again.

Vivekananda

If you serve Truth for many years without swerving from it, people will be convinced by everything you say. Thus you will confer the greatest blessing on the masses, free them from their chains and uplift the whole nation.

Vivekananda

Bring light into the world in plenty! Light, bring light! Light shall shine on all! The task is not ended until all have come to the Creator. Bring light to the poor and still more light to the rich, for their need is greater than that of the poor. Bring light to the ignorant and more light to the learned, for the vanity of learning in our time is great! So bring light to all!

Vivekananda

You can be sure that you will be given heavenly power if you serve Truth and resist every temptation to abandon it. People will not dare to say things in your presence which you do not recognize as truth.

Vivekananda

Only if you can say honestly and with all your heart: Lord, my God! lead me whither Thou wilt—only then can you free yourself from all bondage and be truly free.

Epictetus

Self-control means self-knowledge; self-knowledge means divine consciousness.

Yesudian

Let none resemble the other; yet let each resemble the highest. How can that be done? Let each be perfect in himself.

Goethe

Freedom is nothing but the elimination of ignorance, and ignorance vanishes only if we know the Self.

Vivekananda

You are the infinite, the universe is in you. Know yourself and listen to the voice of your true Self.

Satyakama

Very softly a god speaks in our breast, very clearly he shows us what is to be striven for and what is to be shunned.

Goethe

I believe we carry in us a spark of that eternal light that must shine in the depths of being and which our weak spirit can only descry from afar. To cause this spark in us to become a flame and realize the divine in us is our highest duty.

Goethe

The best does not become clear through words. The spirit moving us to act is the highest.

Goethe

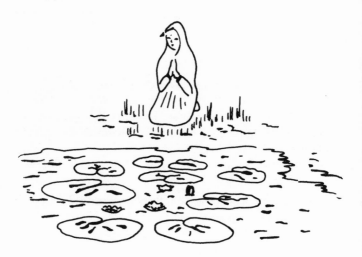

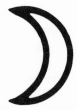

MONDAY
The Power of the Moon

The power of the moon is the natural energy which enables the spirit to embody itself in matter. Just as Nature reflects the creative power of God by bringing forth a million living creatures as the visible material world, so the moon reflects the light of the sun; and thus lunar power, manifested as motherhood, gives back the creative generative power of the male in the birth of the child. That is why the power of the moon, as the representative of Nature, is the inner power of motherhood, of growth, of reflection and of imagination, for imagination is also the embodiment—the reflection—of ideas in pictorial form.

Just as the moon reflects the light of the sun untinctured by alien colors, so should you, O noble-born one, manifest the divinity of your higher self untinctured by the characteristics of your tiny ego.

China

Each newborn child brings the message that God has not yet lost his trust in man.

Tagore

Your outer world is the exact reflection of your inmost being. The perfect body is the faithful image of the perfect soul.

Maharishi

If a woman is capable of giving birth to human beings, what is there in this world she cannot do? Involuntarily man bows down before this holy motherhood to obtain her blessing.

Yesudian

He who regards woman with the eyes of lust has not yet outgrown the state of grossness. Only he who sees the mother in her has risen from the animal and human to the divine plane.

Yesudian

The body is only the outer sheath of the spirit. It must do what the spirit dictates.

Vivekananda

M
o
n
d
a
y

God can become tangible reality only in man.

Ramakrishna

Only if a man's eyes are pure can he see the eternal
mother in woman. Only then does she lavish her grace
upon him.

Yesudian

As a mother lights a lamp in order to make light in a
room, so let the light of truth be kindled in my heart
through your words, O Master.

Yesudian

The child asked: "Mother dear, wake me when I am
hungry." The mother replied: "My dear, hunger itself will
wake you when it is time."

Ramakrishna

The world can be good and pure only if our life is good
and pure. Be pure and calm, the fretful soul can never
reflect the Self.

Vivekananda

The limits of our body are a hollow form. Soul and spirit
must pour into it, shatter it, and constantly enlarge and
reshape it until there is accord between their infinity and
the finite limited form.

Aurobindo

A mother's standing is the highest in the world, for as a mother one learns and practises the greatest selflessness. Only the love of God is greater than the love of a mother.

Vivekananda

Imagine reality to yourself. And then what you imagine will become reality.

E. Haich

The soul is sexless. Why should it lower itself through the imagination of one sex? Whoever wants to be a complete yogi must abandon the idea of one sex.

Vivekananda

The understanding is like the moon. It receives the light of consciousness from the Self, which is like the sun. And so if the Self begins to shine, the understanding becomes unnecessary, like the moon when the sun has risen.

Maharishi

God and Nature are like a boy and girl at play and in love. They hide and run away from each other so that they can chase, seek and catch each other.

Aurobindo

Man was born in order to subdue the great mother, Nature. Not in order to follow her!

Vivekananda

M
o
n
d
a
y

The senior teacher is ten times more honorable than the junior teacher. The father is one hundred times more honorable than the senior teacher. But the mother is one thousand times more honorable than the father.

India

Freedom is the law of Being in its unlimited unity, it is the secret master of Nature. Servitude is the law of love in Being which voluntarily submits in order to serve the interplay of its forms in diversity.

Aurobindo

Do not build splendid edifices in the imagination which ultimately dissolve and leave nothing behind.

Sabhapatti

You are immortal spirits, free spirits, blessed and eternal. You are neither matter nor body. Matter is your servant; you are not the servant of matter.

Vivekananda

By both the infertility and monotony of sheer stillness, Nature shows that what she wants from us is the play of activities on the firm basis of rest. God plays eternally and never grows weary.

Aurobindo

Self-realization alone is true birth.

Maharishi

M
o
n
d
a
y

Through pain and sorrow Nature reminds the soul that
the pleasures it enjoys are only faint intimations of the
true bliss of existence.

Aurobindo

If the moon is full—then it will wane!

China

Body or matter are the expression of Nature. The aim is
to master them and make them a tool that embodies and
expresses the Self, the Divine in us.

Yesudian

Bodily form which encloses and protects the spiritual so
that each can manifest its particular mode of action is
called Nature.

Dsuang Dai

Man is enamored of the limits of his physical existence yet
at the same time yearns for the freedom of his unlimited
spirit and his immortal soul.

Aurobindo

The restlessness and early exhaustion of our active being
and its instruments are Nature's signs that stillness is our
true foundation and commotion a sickness of the soul.

Aurobindo

"Love thy neighbor as thyself," for every man is thine own image. Thou art that. Ta tvam asi.

E. Haich

Neither God can cease to bend down to Nature nor man to strive upwards to Deity. That is the eternal relationship between the finite and the infinite. If they seem to turn away from each other, it is only to meet again at a profounder level.

Aurobindo

Absolute mastery of Nature and nothing else must be the aim. We must be master over Nature and not her slave.

Vivekananda

Life brings a man fruit but it seldom hangs and greets us from the bough as gay and red as an apple.

Goethe

The animal is man, clad in fur and on all fours. The worm is man, it writhes and creeps towards the unfolding of its humanity. Even the undifferentiated forms of matter are the incipient body of man. All things are man.

Aurobindo

Even if books and written works reflect a great deal of knowledge, true wisdom can come only from ourselves.

Yesudian

M
o
n
d
a
y

"Unhappy is the earth that lies fallow for a long time. It is like a fine-bodied woman that has long remained childless." Work on your body which is your portion of the earth with the power of the spirit and it will bear you the divine child: your self-awareness in the divine Self.

E. Haich

A mother is a blessing to everyone in his need. He who has a mother has a protectress, and he who has none is without a protectress.

Mahabharata

Truly blessed is the man to whom woman is the representative of God's motherhood.

Vivekananda

Nature is waiting only to be tamed and made to work. Only if our senses are reined in like horses do man's abilities become manifest. Until then he creeps on all fours.

Yesudian

There is nothing in man that he must tame so much as his imagination, the most versatile and at the same time the most dangerous of all the gifts of the human mind.

Herder

Where women live in sorrow, the family soon perishes. Where women live in happiness, the family always thrives.

China

What you do not leave free will never grow. Give man the light of freedom. That is the only condition of growth.
Vivekananda

Unification is the great secret of Nature. Unification determines all things. The closer a being draws towards unification, the more perfect will this being grow. This is a proposition which everyone understands.
Eckartshausen

A chaste woman who regards every man, save her husband as a child and behaves like a mother to all men, will, through her purity, exercise such power that every man, be he never so brutal, must feel the atmosphere of holiness in her presence.
Vivekananda

Work and worship bring you back to your own nature.
Vivekananda

Always take the shortest path! Nature points to it. Your acts and talk will then be straight and right. This intention alone liberates from all frustrations and troubles, from calculation and hypocrisy.
Marcus Aurelius

Man at first seeks blindly and does not even know that he is seeking his divine Self; for he starts from the darkness of material Nature, and even when he begins to see, he is dazzled for a long time by the growing light within himself. And God's response to his seeking is also veiled: He seeks and enjoys man's blindness like the little hands of a child groping for its mother.

Aurobindo

Neither body nor mind must be master over us. We must remember that the body belongs to us and not we to the body.

Vivekananda

Just as sun and moon cannot be reflected in muddy water, so the Almighty cannot be reflected in a heart that is muddied by the idea of "I and my."

Ramakrishna

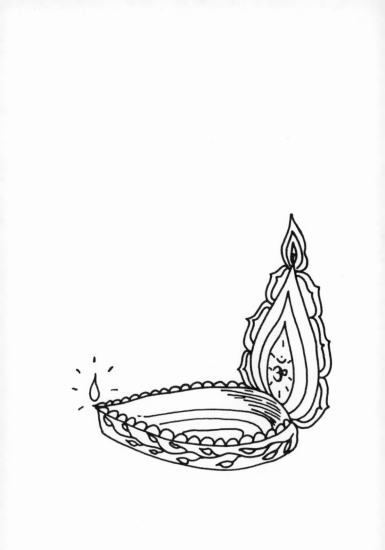

TUESDAY
The Power of Mars

The power of Mars is the creative generative energy which, in a struggle against the natural resistance of the Eternal Feminine, masters, penetrates and fertilizes it. The creative energy of God is manifested as generative power through the body, through the flesh, and serves to maintain the species. Thus in its earthly manifestation Martian power appears as willpower, impulsiveness, courage and daring in making a decision, in engaging in a struggle, as brute muscular strength with which to fight and conquer, and as sexual energy with which to possess and fertilize the Feminine once conquered.

He who does not dissipate his energies but masters them will become the leader of men. He radiates his powerful generative influence on the crowd and strides ahead. His thoughts will penetrate to the very heart of the human community like generative power and fire men and women to deeds of courage and strength. His words will arouse. His deeds will make free. And his very touch will transform a man.

Yesudian

The Self will not be attained by the weak. If there is no vigor in the body and in the soul, the Self cannot be realized. First you must build up your body with good, nutritious food, for only in this way will your soul also be strong. The soul is the finer part of your body. You must store up great energy in your body and in your soul.

Vivekananda

Your own will is the only thing that will answer your prayers.

Vivekananda

This strenuous age needs men with iron wills. Only the man can survive it who knows what he wants.

Yesudian

There is one virtue above all others: the constant striving upwards, the struggle with oneself, the insatiable demand for greater purity, wisdom, goodness and love.

Goethe

EQUANAMINITY CONSERVES PRANA

The man who gives way to anger or hate or any other passion cannot work, for he simply dissipates his forces and does nothing useful. The quiet, forgiving, just and equable man accomplishes the greatest work. He does not lose energy.

Peaceful warrior meets force—not with force but wisdom

Vivekananda

Whenever the animal in man awakes, he is seized by the spirit of destruction and he leaves behind the traces of decay. Whenever the divine in man awakes, he reveals the best in himself and raises the world around him to a higher level.

Yesudian

Spiritual energies are sublimated sexual energies. Sexual energies are materialized spiritual energies.

E. Haich

We conquer the cosmos, we fight against the elements. We are victorious over enemies. But there still remains the greatest of all victories to be won: over the unknown man—over ourselves!

Yesudian

Be cautious—and daring!   *Yoga mimamsa*

The spiritual man is like a giant among dwarfs. He is dependent on no earthly power but only on his immortal spirit, and that is what makes him invincible on earth.

Yesudian

I was born a fighter, so let me fight to the end, with the sword of fearlessness in my right hand and the shield of judgment in my left.

Yesudian

Fools fear fate. The hero overcomes it.

Yesudian

Power cannot be manifested where weakness is. Be what you are! Your true nature is power.

Vivekananda

He who lives must die: so die after a worthy life, as a hero and not as a vanquished slave.

Yesudian

The more circumstances are hostile to you, the more your inner strength will be manifest.

Vivekananda

Let me die on the battlefield of life, after all enemies have been defeated and passions overcome, when hate has changed into love, disdain into understanding, and pride into dignified self-assurance.

Yesudian

No limits are set to the might of man, neither to the power of the word nor to that of the spirit.

Vivekananda

I take no orders but I myself give orders and my armies owe me obedience. The greatest among my warriors are called: "Fearlessness" and "Strength."

Yesudian

The valued man has no quarrels
The quarrelsome man has no value.

Lao-Tse

The power of the spirit comes from control of the energies in the body. The aim is to gather up the forces of the body and to transform them into spiritual and intellectual energies. The greatest danger lies in dissipating the energies of the body in intemperate and injudicious pleasures, in this way we lose the original strength of the spirit.

Vivekananda

The true sign of strength is controlled action.

Yesudian

The man who overcomes himself frees himself from the power that binds all creatures.

Goethe

A nation perishes unless it brings forth the right men for the fulfillment of its task. Bring forth strong men, powerful and honest to the very marrow. Bring forth courageous men. Bring forth men of firm faith. For these are the salt of the nation and the foundation of the great national edifice which will be shelter, protection and inspiration for future generations.

Yesudian

Let even the brute strength of man that uproots mountains rest at bottom upon the spirit!

Japan

The strong man understands strength. The elephant understands the lion, not the rat. How can we understand the great ones of mankind unless we are like them?

Vivekananda

The conquerors are kings; the conquered are bandits.

China

The whole secret of existence is to have no fear. Do not fear what is to become of you and depend on no one. You are free only when you refuse all aid.

Vivekananda

Be bold! Be fearless! Be free! Awake! Arise! and march forward!

Yesudian

God created the earth as a battlefield and filled it with the ringing footsteps of warriors and the cry of strife and struggle. Will you wrest from Him His peace without paying the price he has set for it?

Aurobindo

Cast off your sleep, your sloth! Cast off the prisoner's chains! Cast off your weakness, cast off your woe! He is bound who thinks he is bound and free who thinks he is free.

Yesudian

Have no weakness in you, not even in the face of death. Neither regret past deeds nor brood over them. Do not recall your good deeds. Be free. The weak, the fearful, the ignorant will never attain the Self.

Vivekananda

Your weak eye, O immortal one, strengthened with telescopes and microscopes shows you unknown things: what will the eye of your spirit discover for you when you have learned the art of strengthening it?

Yesudian

Cowards and the faint-hearted can accomplish nothing in life. They come and go from life to life, complaining and sighing. The earth needs heroes! That is the truth without doubt. Be a hero! Say continually: "I have no fear! I am not afraid!" Say that to everyone: "Have no fear! Be fearless!"

Vivekananda

There are no bad energies, only energies badly used.

E. Haich

What we need is a faith that forms people. We need men! Men with muscles of iron and nerves of steel.

Vivekananda

How do all the energies of the universe originate? Through struggle, contest, conflict! Supposing all the particles of matter were continuously in equilibrium, would there then be any creative process at all?

Vivekananda

Above all things be strong and manly! Physical weakness is at the root of at least one third of our unhappiness.

Vivekananda

The sum total of the forces of joy and pain that are at work here on earth always remains the same. We simply shift these forces from one side to the other and then back again but the sum total will remain the same.

Vivekananda

A four-horse carriage can either hurtle downhill out of control or the coachman can rein in the horses. Which is the sign of greater strength: to let the horses run or to hold them back?

Vivekananda

Have the courage to come to the truth, even if the way lies through hell.

Vivekananda

T
u
e
s
d
a
y

Never lose faith in your own strength, and you can do anything in this world. Do not weaken! All strength is yours!

Vivekananda

Pain is a holy angel and through him men have become greater than through all the joys of the world.

Stifter

Only the strong are sorely tempted, so that they may become stronger.

Saretni

Do not expect help from others because by so doing you will be making debts. Believe in yourself, you need no help! You will find all the strength you need in yourself.

Yesudian

It is better to die on the battlefield than live vanquished.

China

He who has a will of his own to impress on things will never let things overwhelm him.

Nietzsche

The will is stronger than anything else. Everything must yield to the will, for it comes from God. A pure and strong will is all-powerful.

Vivekananda

Above all things be strong, be manly! I have respect even for the wicked man if he is manly and strong. One day his strength will take him so far that he will give up his wickedness and even desist from all wicked and selfish actions; and that will bring him to Truth in the end.

Vivekananda

When a cultured man feasts on the art and poetry of the past, he will never be able or willing to dispel completely the illusion that those who created this greatness were happy at the time. In fact they saved the ideal of their times only at the cost of great sacrifice and in their daily life fought the fight we all fight. Only for us do their creations have the appearance of youth saved and garnered.

Jacob Burckhardt

Look back upon yourself from the amoeba to the human being. Who did all that? Your own will. Can you deny then that it is all-powerful? What has raised you so high can raise you still higher. What you must have is character, strengthening of the will.

Vivekananda

Irresolution and despondency do not arise from soreness of distress but from faintness of heart.

St. Chrysostom

If your goal is great and your resources small, act nevertheless. Only through action will your resources grow.

Aurobindo

T
u
e
s
d
a
y

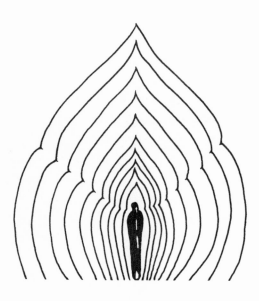

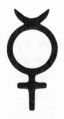

WEDNESDAY
The Power of Mercury

The power of Mercury is the bridge or link between the Divine and the personal Self, between spirit and body. It is the power of thought. Its tool is the understanding, its weapons are the spoken and written word. The power of Mercury helps us to attain the great goal through learning and teaching, which lead to knowledge.

Embodied forms of thought cohere like drops of water in the sea and in their totality form the external world.

Mahayana philosophy

He who really wants to be a yogi must give up once and for all tasting first one thing and then another. Seize hold of a single idea. Let brain, muscles, nerves, and every part of your body be filled with this idea and give not thought to any other. This leads to success and in this way great minds are formed.

Vivekananda

Things are never bad in themselves; only the way you think about them.

Epictetus

The knowledge yoga exercises bring of the essential nature of things which have both relative and real being leads to liberation from ignorance.

Mahayana philosophy

We should like to know the wave on which we drift in the ocean but we are ourselves the wave.

Jacob Burckhardt

There is a great difference between thinking what others have thought and saying what others have said, and between thinking and saying things for oneself.

Eckartshausen

Independence in thinking is the first mark of freedom. Without it you remain a slave to circumstances.

Vivekananda

Your thinking in spiritual matters should be just as rational as in matters of everyday life. External tasks call for rational thought. The spiritual life calls for a thousandfold measure of rational, exact, and well-founded thinking.

Vivekananda

The understanding is the great negator of the real. Deny the negator!

Vivekananda

The effect of light is infinite; it extends to the understanding and reason.

Eckartshausen

Show an Italian, a Frenchman, an Englishman, and an Arab a rose—through looking at it they will all understand what a rose looks like, but not through the medium of words. Words, then, and not things are the reason why we do not understand one another.

Eckartshausen

There is, however, one impurity which surpasses all impurities, and that is ignorance. Oh, wise man, discard that impurity and be free from all impurities.

Dhammapada

Evil thoughts are originators of disease, for every thought is a little hammer blow on the metal of our body and beats out what we shall be. We are the heirs of all good thoughts in the Universe if we open ourselves to them.

Vivekananda

The greatest gift is the gift of knowledge. The greatest strength is mastery of our thoughts.

Yesudian

You shall first hear about the Self. Hear day and night that you are the Self. Repeat it to yourself day and night until it flows into your veins, until it tingles in each drop of your blood, until it becomes flesh and bone in you. Let your whole body be penetrated by this single ideal: "I am the never-born, the never-dying, the blessed, the all-knowing, almighty, eternally glorious Self!" All your deeds will be glorified, transfigured, deified by the true power of thought. If matter is mighty, then thought is almighty!

Vivekananda

The wind gathers the clouds and the wind drives them away. The understanding creates fetters and the understanding also releases us from them.

Sankaracharya

Go within yourself and from out of your own Self fetch knowledge. You are the greatest book that ever was and ever will be, the infinite custodian of everything that is. All external teaching is vain so long as the inner teacher does not awake. It must cause the book of the heart to open if it is to be of value.

Vivekananda

I am a born pupil. Everything that exists is my master. I learn from everything!

Keshab

The treasure of knowledge is a great fortune from which blood relations can take away nothing, which the thief cannot steal, and however much of it you give away, it never grows less!

India

When humanity learnt to speak, it forgot to think for itself.

Karinthy

No single spoken word has ever been so much use as the many words that have remained unspoken.

Plutarch

Water the Tree of Knowledge and let it grow, but eat fruit only from the Tree of Life.

E. Haich

He who knows every day what he does not know, and knows every month what he knows, is learning seriously.

Lao-Tse

To know that one knows nothing, that is the highest of all. To suppose that ignorance is knowledge brings suffering. Only he who suffers from suffering will be released from suffering. He who is called is free from suffering because he suffers from suffering.

Lao-Tse

One does not speak about what one has.
What one speaks about, one does not have.

Lao-Tse

Fate yields obediently like a bent bow in your hands if you shoot the arrow of right thoughts with it.

Yesudian

He who possesses knowledge, wisdom and discrimination is mature enough to seek the Self.

Sankaracharya

An honest thought can move heaven and earth.

China

Neither breathing nor physical yoga exercises are of any use until you have grasped the idea: "In reality I am nothing but a witness. Nothing can touch me from outside!"

Vivekananda

The body—the form—will be shaped by the thought that underlies it.

Vivekananda

Experience is the only teacher we possess. We can talk and debate for a lifetime and yet not understand a word spoken out of Truth until we have experienced it on ourselves.

Vivekananda

The way to destroy ignorance is unceasing practice in discrimination.

Vivekananda

He who is indifferent to the calumny of others vanquishes all things.

Mahabharata

How, When? and Where?—The gods give no reply!
Keep to Because and do not question Why?

Goethe

Curb your tongue to know your thoughts.
Curb your thoughts to know your true Self.

Yesudian

Arise and be free! Know that every thought that weakens you and every word that weakens you is the only real evil in this world. Everything that weakens a man, everything

Wednesday

that arouses fear in him, is the only evil that he should meticulously avoid.

Vivekananda

From childhood onwards fill your brain with positive, strong, useful thoughts. Take in only thoughts of this kind and none that are weakening and crippling. Say to yourself: "I am the Self, the ever-free, immortal Self!" Let it sound in your brain like a song day and night, and on your deathbed declare: "I am the Self!"

Vivekananda

It is the misfortune of the unreasonable to take what is not unreasonable to be unreasonable.

Lu Bu We

Through breath control we achieve thought control, through thought control we enter the original paradisiacal state.

Maharishi

How can I control the understanding?—When the true Self has been realized, there is no longer any understanding to control.

Maharishi

I do not want a teacher who influences me. But I want a teacher who teaches me not to let myself be influenced.

Yesudian

W
e
d
n
e
s
d
a
y

Drive superstition from your brain. Be bold. Recognize the truth and practise it. However distant be the goal, no matter, awake, arise and do not cease until you have reached the goal.

Vivekananda

The men who stand highest are quiet, still and unknown. These are men who really know the power of thought. They know that even if they were shut in a cave, and there thought only five true thoughts and then died, these five thoughts would survive through all eternity. For truly such thoughts will penetrate mountains, cross seas, and wander over the whole earth. They will enter deep into human hearts and brains and will awaken men and women.

Vivekananda

If the shoes are right, no one thinks of the feet. If the belt is right, no one thinks of the hips. If the heart is right, there is no pro and no contra. If the understanding about things is right, there is no inner vacillation and no subjection to outside influence.

Dsuang Dai

Do you know the true meaning of the word Buddha?—It means that by constant pondering over the consciousness one becomes consciousness itself.

Ramakrishna

He who knows the doctrines by heart but does not practise them is like a man who lights a lamp and closes his eyes.

Eckartshausen

The wisdom of most scholars is confined to what others have thought and said.

Eckartshausen

Knowledge that does not grow every day will dwindle daily.

China

Learning is like rowing upstream. If you make no progress, you drift back.

China

Thinking is neither the cause nor the essence of being but it is the instrument of becoming: I become what I see in myself; everything thought suggests to me I can do; everything it manifests to me I can become. On this man should base his unshakeable self-confidence because the Divine dwells in him.

Aurobindo

If we speak to a worldling, we can see that his heart is filled with worldly thoughts and wishes as the crop of a pigeon is filled with grain.

Ramakrishna

Doctrine is like a raft that carries you to the opposite bank. But who would be so foolish as to carry the raft on his shoulders and go on dragging it over dry land simply because it was useful on the water.

Buddha

Wisdom is a treasure that accompanies its owner everywhere.

China

Once we have left knowledge behind us, we shall have knowledge of the real nature of things; Thinking was the means; thinking is the barrier.

Aurobindo

If you cannot compose yourself to thought continually, then compose yourself from time to time, at least twice a day, in the morning and the evening. In the morning form your resolution, and in the evening consider how you have conducted yourself today in thought, word, and deed.

Thomas a Kempis

Do not speak much but feel the spirit within you . . . This is knowledge, all the rest is ignorance.

Vivekananda

Life is only a bridge; do not build a house on it.

China

Wednesday

What does it matter to you what your forefathers thought or what others think today? What matters is what you think; independent, fearless thoughts born of the wealth of your own experience.

Yesudian

The thought of anything imperfect creates an imperfection. Only thoughts of strength and perfection can heal this.

Vivekananda

We are what our own thoughts have made us; so pay heed to what you think.

Vivekananda

The field of doing and action is the proper domain and inheritance of human understanding. It seldom goes wrong when active.

Goethe

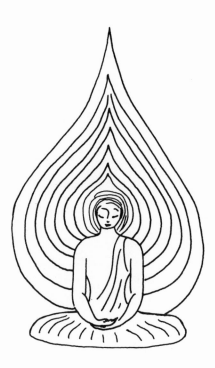

♃

THURSDAY
The Power of Jupiter

The power of Jupiter is the vision of the spirit. The eyes of the body have the ability to perceive the rays of light that stream into them. The spiritual eye on the other hand does not see what enters it but, conversely, radiates visual power from out of itself onto what it wants to see, and does not look at the surface but penetrates what it gazes upon, pierces it, and sees not the outside but the true inner essence of everything. On the material level the power of Jupiter infuses the contemplation of the experienced and wise man who obtains his knowledge and insight not from what he learns or studies but from his inner spiritual vision. Inner vision leads to the true religion and true faith which transcend all false thoughts and all superstition, which know no sects and contradictions—to the one inner faith in God.

Do you long for God?—Very well! Seek him in man. Man is the highest manifestation of God.

Ramakrishna

It is not belief in a supreme Being, nor its denial, but only one's own endeavours towards right living and self-acquired spiritual development that can lead to liberation.

Buddha

It makes a great difference whether I say "Food, food" or eat it, whether I say "Water, water" or drink it. We cannot hope to achieve realization simply by repeating the word "God, God"; we must strive for realization and practise it.

Vivekananda

In eating, sleeping, fearing and begetting, man and animal are alike. Only through religious practice does man raise himself above the animal. This being so, how can he be other than an animal if he is without religion.

Eckartshausen

Sorrow comes from spiritual short-sightedness. The cure is faith founded on wisdom.

Brunton

Wisdom frees from doubt, virtue frees from suffering, resolution frees from fear.

Confucius

Ignorance is the worst of evils. Only wisdom helps to overcome it. And this is achieved only through indefatigable effort.

Eckartshausen

Scholars in our century have forgotten that theory owes its existence to practice and that Nature existed before there were rules.

Eckartshausen

You, whose soul is intended for receptivity to higher things, you, man and brother, you will understand me. And you whose soul is not so attuned, you are not meant to understand me.

Eckartshausen

A man is not wise simply because he talks a great deal. He who is calm, free from hate, and fearless is called a wise man.

Dhammapada

There are no fetters like the fetters of illusion, no power like the power that yoga gives us; there is no higher friend than wisdom and no greater enemy than selfishness.

Gheranda Samhita

One can lead a family life without fear if one possesses wisdom and devoutness. It is easy to walk on thorns if one wears shoes.

Ramakrishna

Control your speech through the power of the mind, control your mental power through your capacity for discrimination, control this ability through the individual will, merge individuality with the infinite, absolute Self and attain the highest peace.

Sankaracharya

According to the old religion, an atheist is someone who does not believe in God. The new religion says: an atheist is someone who does not believe in himself.

Vivekananda

If the wise man has driven out vanity with all seriousness, he rises to the highest level of wisdom and looks down from there upon the fools. Serenely he looks upon the mass of men bent under care like one who .ooks down from the mountain peak upon those left behind in the valley.

Dhammapada

The wise man was asked: "Whom do you love more, your brother or your friend?"
The wise man answered: "I love my brother if he has become my friend!"

Old Jewish Wisdom

God is in all men, but not all men are in God. That is why they suffer!

Ramakrishna

Those who fight their way through errors to truth: these are the wise!
Those who persist in error are the fools.

Rückert

By raising himself through honesty, abstinence, and self-control, the wise man builds for himself an island which floods cannot inundate.

Buddha

If you want to be wise, be sparing in divulging what you have in your head. Your mouth should be closed, your words prudent, and regard your lips as the very greatest treasure of all.

Babylonian Wisdom

The alligator has such a thick and scaly armour that no weapon can easily pierce it.—Similarly you can preach religion to a worldling and it will find no entry in his heart.

Ramakrishna

Knowledge of God keeps pace with faith. Where there is little faith, great knowledge will be sought in vain.

Ramakrishna

He who has faith has everything, and if it is lacking, he lacks everything.

Ramakrishna

The wise man masters his sense and in his heart becomes one with the infinite, all-knowing and all-pervasive Lord. Only he who separates the eternal from the transient exercises spiritual discipline. Great is the glory of the Being that shines with its own light, of the sublime reality in us.

Upanishads

Every sect has its truth, and every truth has its sect.

China

Religions vary but there is only one single God. God is like water that fills different vessels, and in each vessel the vision of God takes the shape of the vessel. Yet He is One.

Vivekananda

It would not be worth becoming seventy years old if all the wisdom of the world were foolishness before God.

Goethe

He who has recognized God, casts off all fetters, and with his vanished suffering, he sheds birth and death.

Upanishads

The wise man does not alter even in distress. The base man loses his temper.

Confucius

The wise man is peace-loving but he knows no compromises. The ordinary man makes compromises but he is never peace-loving.

Confucius

Religion originates from the power of realization. It is not the number of doctrines or philosophies that is of great value but only what you are and what you have realized.

Vivekananda

The wise man strives in all seriousness and with a firm resolve to be freed from the bondage of the world as if he wanted to be freed from a disease.

Sankaracharya

He who does not know and knows not that he does not know is a fool, let him be. He who does not know and knows that he does not know, is an ignoramus, teach him. He who knows and does not know that he knows is asleep, wake him. He who knows and knows that he knows is a wise man, follow him.

Koran

Great wisdom has no external form. Valuable things cannot be perfected quickly. Noble notes rarely sound.

Lu Bu We

The wise merchant hides his treasures as if he were poor. The noble-minded man hides his wisdom as if he knew nothing.

Li Gi

Everything truly great on earth grows out of something lowly. The wise man does not think of his greatness and thus becomes great.

Lia Dse

The wise man assesses people by their humanity, others assess them by their deeds, and the stupid by their gifts.

Lu Bu We

Have faith in everything you do. Only to the man who has faith in himself do the doors of all worlds open. Faith is complete reliance on the inner spirit that animates all. Know that you are this spirit. Let your deeds be accompanied by the power of the spirit, whether it be a thought, a word or a deed.

Yesudian

One should believe in what is not yet so that it shall become.

E. Haich

The wise man uses his heart like a mirror. He does not seek things and he does not go out to meet them. What comes to him he picks up in his mirror, but does nothing to keep it there. But it is just this that enables him to be victorious over everything and never be hurt himself.

Dsuang Dai

The correct man easily becomes petty and pedantic. The wise man preserves gravity and dignity but always aims at sensible and useful ends.

Kao Yao

Only the ignoramus becomes angry. The wise man
understands.

India

The good-natured and easy-going man is susceptible to
bad influences. The wise man persists firmly and un-
swervingly in the good.

Kao Yao

Understanding of the skill and dexterity of the hand
serves only to eke out your day. But knowledge, liberation from earthly existence, is not this the only true
wisdom?

Kung Dse

May the day be holy to you; but do not esteem life higher
than any other good, and all goods are deceptive.

Goethe

The noble-minded man is self-assured, without ar-
rogance; the man of low degree is arrogant, without self-
assurance.

Kung Dse

Faith can work wonders whereas vanity and egoism are
the death of man.

Ramakrishna

The wise man who, through faith, devotion and meditation, has recognized the Self and become one with Brahman is free from the wheel of eternal change and released from rebirth, suffering and death.

Upanishads

True artists are the most religious of mortals.

Rodin-Gsell

It is not the purpose of the study of philosophy to learn what others have thought but to learn the truth of things.

Thomas Aquinas

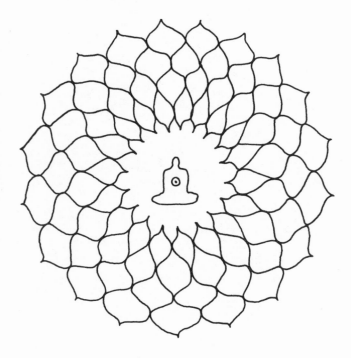

FRIDAY
The Power of Venus

The power of Venus is the motivating force behind the marriage of Nature. In response to this power all creatures, whether plant, animal or man, don their finest array to please the opposite sex, to attract it, and then to celebrate their nuptials together. In its outward form the power of Venus is beauty, harmony, art and love, from animal attraction and lust for possession to the highest impersonal, universal love, at every level throughout the gamut of creation's manifestation.

The great law is Love. It is the efficacious force, the means of assimilation, the chain of unification.

Eckartshausen

There is no vice which does not originate in a withdrawal from love. There is no virtue which is not rooted in love.

Eckartshausen

No creature can approach the Godhead unless it resembles it. And as the Godhead is Love, so resemblance to it comes about through Love. He who withdraws from Love also withdraws from God.

Ramakrishna

Let yourself be linked to everything, whether above or below you, near or far, visible or invisible, with unlimited love, and let no hostile feeling or the desire to kill arise in you against any creature. Live in this consciousness, wherever you stand and walk, sit and lie, until your last breath. Live and have your being in the Spirit of God and you shall find your joy in Him.

Vedanta philosophy

It is not love that makes blind but the craving for possession. Men are blinded by sensual desires. True love frees from that craving and gives us eyes to see.

Ramakrishna

One should not speak of love but act out of love and live in love.

Ramakrishna

Love is love's own reward!   *E. Haich*

Learning and cleverness are the conscious and often presumptuous wisdom of the thoughts. But love is the unconscious wisdom of the whole man.

Wöhrmüller

If we have left joys behind, we shall have blessedness. Desire was the means; desire is the barrier.

Aurobindo

He who loves others and is not loved in turn, let him examine his attitudes to his fellow men.

Mong Dse

Against great merits in others there is no remedy but love.
Goethe

In a union of beauty and ugliness, beauty always triumphs in the end: in obedience to a divine law Nature invariably returns to the better, it strives ceaselessly towards perfection.

Rodin-Gsell

Every one can create true happiness for himself only by making himself independent of fate through his feelings.
W. von Humboldt

Every one who wants to call himself an "artist" legitimately must express the whole truth of Nature, not only its outer but above all its inner truth.

Rodin-Gsell

Pure knowledge and pure love are ultimately one. Pure knowledge leads to the same goal as pure love.

Ramakrishna

Artists and thinkers are like a lyre which has infinitely delicate and plaintive notes. And the vibrations which the spirit of each age coaxes from it awake a response in all other mortals.

Rodin-Gsell

For the man who merits the name of "artist" everything in Nature is beautiful because his eyes, which take in every external truth undaunted, can read there effortlessly, as if in an open book, every inner truth.

Rodin-Gsell

Speak of music only to a musician!

China

Children's love moves heaven and earth.

China

He who cannot love does not know how to live like a human being.

Lavater

To understand the love of your parents you must yourself raise children.

China

Just as the tiger devours other animals, so love devours all the "arch enemies" of mankind such as sensual desire, passion, envy and anger.

Ramakrishna

Plunge deep into the sea of divine love. Fear not! It is the sea of immortality.

Ramakrishna

He in whom the glories of love are manifested attains God at once. What are the glories of love?— Discernment, dispassion, tenderness for all living things, services to good people and joy in fellowship with them, truthfulness. . . . all these.

Ramakrishna

What is the new thing that we still have to perfect?— Love! For so far we have succeeded only with hate and complacency.

Aurobindo

Love is the ground tone, joy is the harmony, power is the melody, knowledge is the player, the infinite Universe is the composer and the audience. We hear the tuning of the instruments which is as violent as the harmony will be tremendous; but we shall reach the fugue of divine beatitudes.

Aurobindo

Now there remain Faith, Hope and Charity, these three; but the greatest of these is Charity.

1 Cor. XIII, 13

He alone finds God who longs for Him as a loving wife longs for her husband, as a worldling longs for earthly joys, and as a miser longs for his hoarded gold.

Ramakrishna

True love does not mean watering weeds. If you do not allow yourself to lie, to steal, and to commit other sins against unity then do not allow them to your neighbour out of a false sense of charity.

E. Haich

To enter the valley of love, one must plunge wholly into fire. Yes, one must become fire oneself, for otherwise one cannot live there. He that truly loves must resemble fire, his countenance aflame, burning and impetuous like fire.

Farid ud-Din Attar: The Talk of the Birds

In this valley love is the fire, and its smoke is reason. When love comes, reason flees away in haste. Reason cannot live together with the frenzy of love, love has nothing to do with human reason.

Farid ud-Din Attar: The Talk of the Birds

Love is the law of the Divine, the commandment that the Divine laid in the heart of man. It is the bond that unites all creatures. The urge to unification arises from it. To grow similar is its nourishment.

Eckartshausen

Just open your eyes: everything is beautiful!

Thoma

Do not confuse true, impersonal charity with weakness! True love is firm and hard. If we want to be a pillar among men that gives the weak and vacillating security and stability, then we must be as hard as stone.

E. Haich

Love knows no reward. Love is always there for love's sake.

Confucius

What is true and good is beautiful,
What is beautiful and true is good,
What is beautiful and good is true.

Lorant Hegedüs

Supreme love and supreme perfection consist of supreme concord, supreme harmony.
This harmony resembles the notes of music which consist of endless gradations and yet each note from the lowest to the highest stands in relation to the whole.

Eckartshausen

Talent without diligence is not art; diligence without talent is not art; talent and diligence—is art!

E. Haich

Love is ceaselessly active; its attribute is a constant endeavour to bring forth its like; herein lies the reason for creation—the calling forth of creatures—our ordainment.

Eckartshausen

The nature of perfection and harmony excludes every imperfection and every disharmony; it therefore lies in the nature of the Supreme Being that only desire for harmony can lead to Supreme Love—to God.

Eckartshausen

What is the greatest art?—and what is the easiest thing to do? The greatest art is self-control, and the easiest thing to do is criticize our neighbours.

E. Haich

On looking at what is in the mirror in front of you, think of what is behind it.

Wu Wang

Be as free from vanity as the shriveled leaf which the storm drives in front of it.

Ramakrishna

It is not for the husband's sake that the wife loves the husband, but rather, she loves him for the sake of the Self, because she loves the Self.

No man loves a woman for the woman's sake, but because he loves the Self, he loves the woman.

No one loves the children for the children's sake, but because he loves the Self he loves the children.

No one loves an object for the object's sake, but rather, we love it for the sake of the Self.

That is why this Self must be heard, considered and meditated on. If this Self has been heard, if this Self has been seen, if this Self has been realized, then all this you know.

Vedanta philosophy

If you play the flute, you must learn the fingering the composer prescribes for you; to sing a song harmoniously, you must raise or lower your voice according to the written score. In just the same way you must set to work if you want to play the grand harmonica of Nature: unless you follow these rules, you will be a wretched performer and the wise man will stop his ears against the din.

Eckartshausen

The Bible teaches: "Love thy neighbor as thyself." That means that you must first be able to love—and to forgive—yourself before you can love your neighbor aright.

E. Haich

Tell me, where doth grow the seed
Of the herb "Forgetfulness?"
It grows in every human heart
Devoid of lovingness.

Sosei Fu

And though I have the gift of prophecy, and understand all mysteries, and all knowledge; and though I have all faith, so that I could remove mountains, and have not charity, I am nothing.

1 Corinthians XIII, 2

A new commandment I give unto you, That ye love one another; as I have loved you, that ye also love one another.

John 13, 34

Because for Goethe love is the highest form of the spirit, he cannot conceive of God, as the epitome of all spirituality, other than as the fullness of love.

Albert Schweitzer

We see love everywhere in Nature. Everything that is good, great and majestic in society comes from love; everything in society that is wicked, demonic even, originates from aberrant feelings of love . . . Thus love manifests itself, this ardent longing of two beings to become one, and perhaps even the longing of all beings to pour themselves into a single one, everywhere, differing according to circumstances, more or less pure, but nevertheless as the one love.

Vivekananda

Oh man, whatever you love that you will be changed into. You will become God, if you love God, and the earth if you love the earth.

Angelus Silesius

In a conflict between the heart and the head, follow the heart.

Vivekananda

Expansion means life, love is expansion. Love is therefore the only law of life. He who loves, lives.

Vivekananda

The Tree of Life blossoms only for the light of heart.

Ernst Moritz Arndt

Piety can and should be cultivated in a good temper; one can and should do arduous but necessary work in a good temper, and indeed even die in a good temper; for everything loses its value by being done or suffered in a bad temper and ill humor.

Kant

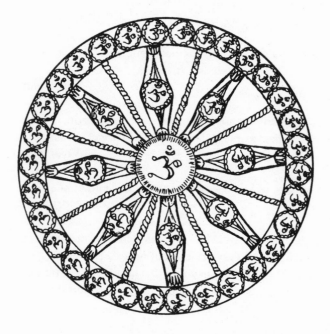

♄

SATURDAY
The Power of Saturn

The fact that matter exists at all is due to the cooling, contracting and rigidifying effect of the power of Saturn, but the same power also makes liberation from matter possible. For spiritualization can only come about through contraction—concentration. That is why in the Bible the power of Saturn is the key with which Peter—the rock— opens or closes heaven to us. The power of Saturn is manifested on the earthly as well as on the spiritual and intellectual plane. Hardness and firmness are qualities of matter and also of man, who can be hard or firm in his mind. Thus the power of Saturn is manifested as contraction in materialization and crystallization on the material level—as thrift, covetousness or parsimony on the spiritual—and as concentration of thought on the intellectual level. Additional manifestations of Saturn are steadfastness, perseverance, fidelity, renunciation, and asceticism, but also transience and death.

Be steadfast and determined! Character means the crystallization of our best qualities. The expression of your true nature, the Divine, comes from the control and concentration of your best powers.

Turyananda

Only through steadfastness and fidelity in our present state do we become worthy of the higher stage of a subsequent state and capable of entering it, whether it be temporal here or eternal there.

Goethe

One proof of the steadiness of the spirit, is the steadiness of the gaze. As soon as the spirit has become steady, the gaze will become steady too. Uncertainty of gaze and movement disappear completely.

Turyananda

Learn concentration and apply it in every way. Thus you lose nothing. He who has the whole also has the parts.

Vivekananda

The secret of the extraordinary human being is in most instances nothing but persistence, be it in the love of God, the love of man, in the pursuit of rightly conceived aims, in striving for perfection.

Gillen

The yogi retires into solitude because he can no longer tolerate loneliness between human beings.

E. Haich

We suffer because we are removed from our center. If we know who we are and return to the center, we shed suffering.

Brunton

What we do today creates our future; as the shadow follows the body so we are followed by the law of fate. Each is forced to bear the consequences of his actions himself.

Padma-Sambhava

Allah will guard your camel but first tie it to a tree.

Koran

The world thinks that the yogi is a man of self-denial who renounces everything that life has to offer. The contrary is true! The yogi wants what is highest of all, he wants life itself—God Himself! He renounces only the transient joys and prefers the eternal ones.

E. Haich

Through renunciation one becomes mature. He who has not learnt renunciation cannot keep pace with the limits of his years.

The Templar

Saturday

Anyone treads the path of Yoga if his activities are combined with concentration, for the latter expands the consciousness.

E. Haich

Two things shalt thou avoid, o wanderer: idle wishes and too much mortification of the body.

Buddha

The desireless state frees us from death, for once wishes and desires cease to pull us down into the material world, the cycle of birth and death ceases for us and we are able to enjoy the eternal freedom of the spirit, free from space and time.

E. Haich

Even in the center of the very greatest cyclone there is absolute stillness.

E. Haich

All worldly things are only a dream in spring. Look upon death as a return home.

Confucius

When you entered this world, o man, the world laughed with joy—but you wept. Now that you are in the world, live in such a way that when the time comes for you to leave this world, the world will weep—but you will depart in laughter.

Tulsi

He who is master of himself through his own power is like the Pole Star; he does not move and the universe revolves round him.

Confucius

Man is enamoured of the fetters of birth, and therefore he is also caught in the corresponding fetters of death. In these chains he demands the complete fulfillment of his Self.

Aurobindo

The noble man knows how to bear misfortune with resolution and dignity. The base-minded man loses control of himself in misfortune.

Confucius

May every gentle nature of the better kind envelop itself in that material hardness which is now indispensable in the struggle with the earthly powers.

Feuchtersleben

There can be no human life without cares, but to live carefree with cares, often indeed with many cares, that is the art of living to which we should be brought up.

Hilty

Immutability in the centre is what determines virtue; is it not even its epitome? Men seldom persist therein.

Confucius

S
a
t
u
r
d
a
y

The soul can really and truly hold fast only to what has truly come from out of ourselves in freedom.

W. von Humboldt

Perseverance is a daughter of strength, obstinacy a daughter of weakness.

Ebner-Eschenbach

Strong men remain true to their nature, whatever unhappy state of life fate may cast them into, their character remains firm and their minds unswerving. Fate can have no power over such men.

Machiavelli

Firmness of character means having felt and withstood the effects of other people on oneself; and for that other people are necessary.

Stendhal

Steadfast is the man who remains in his place; truly does he live who proves himself in death.

Lao-Tse

Yet he is neither unwise nor stupid who after an error picks himself up from his fall instead of persisting defiantly in wrong.

Sophocles

S
a
t
u
r
d
a
y

What are riches to a skinflint who is dirty, wears shabby clothes, always wants to eat very little, and is far more wretched than a poor man?

Ksemendra

Inner greed is not satisfied with money any more than thirst with salt water. The suffering of the greedy is visibly much greater than the suffering of the have-nots.

Ksemendra

The noble man is steadfast in distress. When the inferior man falls on hard times, he becomes defiant.

Confucius

The true man knows no pleasure at being born nor any dread of dying. His entry into the world of physicality was no joy to him and his going hence was without reluctance.

Dsuang Dai

Strength of character shows in observance of the just mean, and it is an essential part of that strength that it should have the just mean as its aim. But wrongdoing is multiform.

Aristotle

The man who truly possesses persistence in treading the path of human life: even if he be stupid, he will become enlightened; even if he be weak, he will become strong.

Dsung Yung

The trials that beset us serve to confirm our faith, to really purify us, and to get rid of the dross. For though we are sinners, the divine influence persists in the world.

Judah ha-Levi

Death is the question that Nature constantly asks life, and her warning that life has not yet found itself. If life were not beset by death, the creature would persist for ever in some imperfect form of life. Persecuted by death it awakes to the idea of the perfect life and seeks its conditions and possibilities.

Aurobindo

Fools rush in pursuit of outwardly directed desires and fall into the open snare of death. But the wise who have recognized immortality as that which abides amidst mutable things have no further desire for them.

Upanishads

Thrift makes man independent, miserliness makes man a slave.

E. Haich

Repayment for good and evil is like the shadow that follows the body.

China

What is generated through procreation is death. But that through which procreation becomes procreation has never yet ceased. What is given shape through design is the mass of things. But that through which design becomes design has never yet come into existence.

Lia Dsi: The True Book

Separation from the body does not mean death to those with knowledge.

Mahabharata

The ordinary mortal, with his soul enslaved to all senses and endowed with a wavering memory, goes to his death through betrayal of himself.

Mahabharata

Today death stands before me, as if someone wanted to see his house again after many years spent in captivity.

Egypt

Two kinds of men torment themselves to no purpose and labour in vain: he who collects money and does not use it, and he who acquires knowledge and does not apply it.

Democritus

The miser's money, which causes uneasiness, trouble, thirst, blindness, and sleeplessness, is not money but a sickness of the heart.

Ksemendra

Time and space, the two great beams on which our spirit is crucified, can only be overcome by concentration.

E. Haich

Life is movement, change, transformation; rigidification is death.

E. Haich

For if ye live after the flesh, ye shall die; but if ye through the spirit do mortify the deeds of the body, ye shall live.

Romans VIII, 13

For to be carnally minded is death; but to be spiritually minded is life and peace.

Romans VIII, 6

He is condemned to darkness who devotes himself to life in the world, and to still greater darkness who dedicates himself solely to devotion. He who lives for earthly things alone must expect other things than he who devotes himself only to devotion, so the wise teach us. But he who combines the two, the worldly with the life of devotion, overcomes death through life in the world and attains immortality through devotion.

Upanishads

. . . And so, for example, death is not fearful but to believe of death that it is fearful, that is what is fearful.

Epictetus

. . . nobody knows of death whether it is not the greatest of goods; but they fear it as if they knew for certain it is the greatest of evils.

Plato

Do not stare at the passage of time, fill it with work, and you will have no reason to complain of the loss of lifetime.

Petrarch

He who has no time also has no eternity.

Old proverb

Contraction means death. Selfishness is contraction. He who is selfish dies.

Vivekananda

To be successful you must have enormous perseverance.

Vivekananda

One must oneself be more persistent than the difficulties. There is no other way out.

Aurobindo

SEXUAL ENERGY AND YOGA

The purpose of this book is to introduce the concept of transmuting the physical, emotional, mental and psychic energies people normally disperse in sexual activity. This process assists in uniting with the higher Self or God. Topics include:

- The Creative Primal Serpent
- Sexual Energy in Its False & True Light
- The Magical Powers of Suggestion
- Hypnosis
- Mediumship
- The Urge For Unity & Its Corruptions
- The Sun Creator & Destroyer of Life
- The Magic Flower

"The Transformation of sexual energy into spiritual, divine, creative power, is the resurrection from death to eternal life."

Description by Elisabeth Haich of her painting on the cover

If we cultivate spiritual awareness and attain the universal consciousness, we acquire mastery over the 7 natural forces which, when harnessed to pull in one direction, can carry us to the goal with incredible swiftness.

The picture symbolizes this state. The figure representing the spirit is standing in the triumphal chariot. One hand is radiating the power which directs the natural forces. In the left hand is held a prayer wheel such as is used in Tibet and which symbolizes unity with the Divine. The horses race with this figure to the goal where we achieve the perfection which Christ intimated to us in the words: "Be ye therefore perfect, even as your Father which is in Heaven is perfect."

ELISABETH HAICH

ISBN: 0-943358-03-5 **15 Illustrations** **Paperback** $5^{1}/_{2} \times 8^{1}/_{2}$
158 Pages **$14.95**

INITIATION
ELISABETH HAICH

Written at the request of her advanced students, *Initiation* is an illuminating autobiography that connects the twentieth century European life of internationally beloved teacher Elisabeth Haich and her lucid memories of initiation into the hidden mystical teachings of the priesthood in ancient Egypt. A compelling story within a story emerges detailing the life experiences that catalyzed her spiritual path.

In an earlier life in ancient Egypt, a young woman is prepared for initiation into the esoteric secrets of the priesthood by the High Priest Ptahhotep, who instructs her step-by-step, consistent with her development, in the universal truths of life. Throughout this extraordinary book, Elisabeth Haich reveals her in depth insights into the subtle workings of karma, reincarnation, the interconnectedness of individual daily life choices and spiritual development Elisabeth Haich shares usually hidden truths that only a few rare individuals in any generation, seek, find and communicate to others, enabling the reader to awaken within the essential understanding necessary to enlighten any life no matter what events manifest.

In twentieth century Europe, from childhood to adulthood, through war and remarkable meetings, she demonstrates the power of turning the searchlight of one's consciousness inward and using every life event towards expanding consciousness.

Initiation is a timeless classic communicated in modern terms inspiring generations of spiritual seekers globally. Whether read as an autobiographical novel unveiling mystical truths or as a unique glimpse into Elizabeth Haich's exceptional journey to initiation, the personal impact on the reader is profound.

To read *Initiation* is to be part of the initiation itself.

ISBN:0-943358-50-7   Paperback   5½x 8½   376 Pages $19.95

SELF HEALING,
YOGA & DESTINY

Elisabeth Haich &
Selvarajan Yesudian

Through her best selling books, such as *Initiation*, Elisabeth Haich has become world famous for her profound understanding of the human soul. The Yoga schools she set up with Selvarajan Yesudian, have become internationally renowned. Designed to reconnect you with the Divine, the concepts in this book explain the attitudes necessary for the path back to one's self. Based on many years personal experience, the authors create an understanding of how to realize the essential source of life.

Learn Elisabeth Haich & Yesudian's personal views on:

- Love
- Suffering
- Destiny
- Illness
- Accidents
- Karma
- Black & White Magic
- Self Healing & Transformation

A wealth of insightful information is contained in this book to help you gain an expanded view of your life and consciousness.

"When we look about us in our daily living, we see how greatly people suffer in the chains they have forged for themselves, even when they are filled with longing for freedom. Is there any way for man to be free? To be free is to be free from the deceptive magic of the material world."

HAICH AND YESUDIAN

ISBN: 0-943358-06-X   Paperback   5½×8½   90 Pages $5.95

WISDOM OF THE TAROT

Wisdom of the Tarot relates the path to higher consciousness through the color, shape and symbolic forms on the twenty-two Tarot cards. Detailed study and meditation of each card may release internally all that is involved with each level encountered on the journey towards the Light. These cards may be used in conjunction with the text or separately for meditation. When studied individually, a card can reveal the necessary steps that need to be taken to actualize one's potential.

Tarot cards, or symbolic representations of the truth have always been used to help man relate not only with the mind, but internally, through the feelings invoked by the colors and forms. The nature of these cards is that they can produce a strong awakening of one's unconscious forces. They are like a spiritual mirror in which we can recognize and examine ourselves. We can then understand that the reasons for our fate lie within ourselves, and changes by the mere fact that we begin to react differently to everything that happens to us. These cards with the text are a valuable key to understand our present state, our past and in a deeper sense, how we create our future. Included within the book are pages of five color Tarot cards.

"Elisabeth Haich has produced a masterly work of initiation into the secrets of life. Out of a deep understanding of being and her own intimate experience of union with her genius, she has illustrated the process by which man becomes man by his insight into the pictures of the twenty two rungs of the ladder of divine ascent, on which each rung is an experience for the next rung in accordance with the individual's plan of life." **DR. EWALT KLIEMKE**

ISBN: 0-943358-01-9   Paperback   6×9   174 Pages $12.50

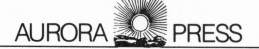

AURORA PRESS

Aurora Press is devoted to pioneering books that catalyze personal growth, balance and transformation. Aurora makes available in a digestible format, an innovative synthesis of ancient wisdom with twentieth century resources, integrating esoteric knowledge and daily life.

Recent titles include:

COMING HOME
Deborah Duda

CRYSTAL ENLIGHTENMENT
Katrina Raphaell

CRYSTAL HEALING
Katrina Raphaell

SILVER DENTAL FILLINGS • THE TOXIC TIMEBOMB
Sam Ziff

AWAKEN HEALING ENERGY THROUGH THE TAO
Mantak Chia

TAOIST SECRETS OF LOVE
Mantak Chia

THE LUNATION CYCLE
Dane Rudhyar

SELF HEALING, YOGA AND DESTINY
Elisabeth Haich

For a complete catalog write:

AURORA PRESS
P.O. BOX 573
SANTA FE NEW MEXICO 87504
Fax 505 982-8321
Email:Aurorep@aol.com